Roger Rios Escobar
Leydis Suárez Ramos
Miralis Cabreja Heredia

EDUCATIONAL INTERVENTION AND ALGORITHMS FOR CUTANEOUS CARCINOMA

Roger Rios Escobar
Leydis Suárez Ramos
Miralis Cabreja Heredia

EDUCATIONAL INTERVENTION AND ALGORITHMS FOR CUTANEOUS CARCINOMA

CUTANEOUS CARCINOMA MAY BE PREDICTABLE

ScienciaScripts

Imprint
Any brand names and product names mentioned in this book are subject to trademark, brand or patent protection and are trademarks or registered trademarks of their respective holders. The use of brand names, product names, common names, trade names, product descriptions etc. even without a particular marking in this work is in no way to be construed to mean that such names may be regarded as unrestricted in respect of trademark and brand protection legislation and could thus be used by anyone.

Cover image: www.ingimage.com

This book is a translation from the original published under ISBN 978-613-9-43947-8.

Publisher:
Sciencia Scripts
is a trademark of
Dodo Books Indian Ocean Ltd. and OmniScriptum S.R.L publishing group

120 High Road, East Finchley, London, N2 9ED, United Kingdom
Str. Armeneasca 28/1, office 1, Chisinau MD-2012, Republic of Moldova, Europe
Printed at: see last page
ISBN: 978-620-8-25993-8

INTERVENTION EDUCATIONAL Y ALGORITHMS FOR CUTANEOUS CARCINOMA

SKIN CARCINOMA MAY BE PREVENTABLE

INDEX

PROLOGUE

Medical and nursing interventions are a framework for achieving knowledge of basal cell carcinoma affecting a given population in order to mitigate the risks of suffering from it or to achieve personal improvement. This leads to the implementation of an educational intervention and algorithm for the comprehensive care of patients with basal cell carcinoma, which includes: sequence of actions, roles of medical and paramedical staff, preventive and therapeutic methods, diagnostic means and the mode of clinical follow-up. A consensus on the theoretical and practical basis of the educational intervention and the use of the algorithm was established using the Delphi variant of the expert method and the health personnel involved in its implementation were trained. A critical analysis of the methods established in the city of nuevitas was carried out, and the national and international literature specialised in Camagüey for the prevention, diagnosis and treatment of the disease was reviewed. The results obtained with the implementation of the educational strategy and the algorithm demonstrated its effectiveness in the integral care of patients with basal cell carcinoma, due to the fact that prevention, early diagnosis, adequate physical examination, correct treatment, notification, periodic clinical follow-up and referral of complicated patients were guaranteed, with the appearance of few complications.

INTRODUCTION

The skin is a layer that covers the human body, protecting it from heat, light, wounds and infections. The human body is made up of very small cells that grow and die in a controlled way. Sometimes these cells keep multiplying, growing out of control, causing abnormal tissue called a tumour. For every two cancers that are diagnosed, about one is skin cancer. Most skin cancers occur after the age of 50, but the damaging effects of the sun begin in childhood, so skin should be protected from an early age to prevent future damage. The most common are non-melanomatous skin cancers, which come in two varieties: basal cell carcinoma (80 %) and squamous cell carcinoma (20 %). (1)

Basal cell carcinoma (BCC) is considered a locally invasive, aggressive and destructive malignant tumour, but rarely metastasises (<0.1%). They are associated with ultraviolet radiation and less frequently with other causes. Mutations of different genes are involved, most notably the Patched tumour suppressor gene on chromosome 9q 22. The clinicopathological appearance and biological behaviour of basal cell carcinoma depend on the interaction between the epithelium and the surrounding stroma. (1,2)

BCC is currently not considered life-threatening for patients, but they represent a major economic impact on health services and lost working days. There is also a psychological impact on the patient's self-esteem as they can appear in visible places on the face. (1, 2,3)

Despite being a malignant tumour, it rarely metastasises. This is why it is also called "Basal cell epithelioma or basalioma", referring to its more benign nature, in relation to other skin cancers where metastasis is frequent, as is the case with squamous cell carcinoma. (1,2, 3,4)

Approximately one out of every two cancers diagnosed is skin cancer. Some countries such as the United States and Colombia report it in the first place of cancer incidence, with low mortality, but significant morbidity. In Europe, 250 000 new cases of epitheliomas appear every year, the most affected countries are Australia and New Zealand, currently considered a serious problem due to its high frequency. (4,5)

In the last 50 years, the countries of Latin America and the Caribbean have undergone demographic and epidemiological changes, which have led to an absolute increase in the number of people suffering from the disease. Cuba is currently one of the Latin American and Third World countries with the highest incidence of non-melanoma skin cancer, with a rate of 55.46 per 100,000 inhabitants. Skin cancer is undoubtedly one of the most common types of cancer. In fact, it accounts for about 50% of all tumours diagnosed annually in the world. In Peru, according to GLOBOCAN 2020, about 1300 new cases of melanoma skin cancer are diagnosed each year. It is therefore important that we all get involved in a culture of prevention that reduces the incidence of this disease and helps to raise awareness about early detection and timely treatment. (6)

In Cuba, the Ministry of Public Health, in its book Prevention, diagnosis and treatment of skin cancer, highlights that it is the most frequent type of cutaneous neoplasia. In 2017, 3956 new cases were diagnosed in the male sex with a crude rate of 70.6 and a world population-adjusted rate of 40.3 per 100 000 inhabitants; as well as 3853 cases in the female sex with a crude rate of 68.3 and a world population-adjusted rate of 38 per 100 000 women.

In 2017, 4817 new cases of squamous cell carcinoma were reported (37.4% of all skin cancers), which was 15% more than reported in 2015. The incidence for males was 2726 cases, a crude rate of 48.7 per 100 000 and a global population-adjusted rate of 27 per 100 000 males. For females, the incidence was lower, with 2091 new cases, a crude rate of 37 per 100 000 and a population-adjusted rate of 18.6 per 100 000 females. (7,8.9)

Statistics indicate that skin cancer is the most frequent cancer(8) and that its incidence is increasing in epidemic proportions worldwide. In Colombia, national rates increased from 23 cases per 100,000 inhabitants in 2008 to 41 cases per 100,000 inhabitants in 2012. Cuba is no exception, with more than 8,000 cases reported between 2011,(9) and 2014, a figure that, according to the 2017 Health Statistical Yearbook,(10) rose to 10,995. In Villa Clara, of the 3 127 tumours with complex prognoses reported in 2017, 1 505 cases were skin neoplasms, (11) which were also found to be the most common type of cancer at this level.This type of neoplasm constitutes a health problem, not only because of its high incidence, but also because of the negative aesthetic, morphological and functional implications of surgical therapy for patients, as well as the high cost of treatment due to the need for re-interventions because of the frequent recurrence of these tumours.· (9)

Health education campaigns lead to early diagnosis and treatment with decreased mortality; this may slow the increase in the frequency of this neoplasm as it is largely dependent on modifiable factors. Skin cancer has not been a public health priority, partly due to low mortality rates of around 1 per 100 000 people per year. However, it has been described how this pathology generates a high public health burden, due to its effect on morbidity and costs to the health system. (10,11)The main pillar that should govern the quality of medical care for patients suffering from non-melanoma skin cancer is to be able to make an early diagnosis, which allows for timely, correct and effective treatment, The treatment will eliminate the malignant neoplastic process of the skin and ensure adequate follow-up of the patient, associated with the pertinent search for other pre-malignant and malignant skin lesions, which often go unnoticed by the patient and which in the medium or long term will lead to the appearance of new skin tumour processes and on the skin, and which will also lead to the appearance of new skin tumours. that rapid action must be taken to avoid future complications. (1,7,9, 10,12)

With this problem identified in the diagnosis of a large number of patients with this disease in Nuevitas who move to the city of Camagüey to receive treatment or to other cities in the country, we are motivated to carry out an educational intervention in relation to knowledge of the disease and an algorithm for the diagnosis and treatment of basal cell carcinoma and the training of health personnel and patients between the ages of 20 and 58 years in the development of practices that contribute to reducing this problem and to improving the quality of life of our population.

Research problem How to achieve knowledge of basal cell carcinoma in the population that generates adequate behaviour and reliability in the appropriate use of specialised treatments?

Research hypothesis: an educational intervention to counteract the effects of basal cell carcinoma in the population, its preventive measures and an algorithm, will allow comprehensive care for these patients.

General objective

To apply an educational intervention and algorithm for the comprehensive care of patients with basal cell carcinoma.

Specific objectives

1- Characterise the carcinoma basal cell carcinoma onpatients belonging to the Francisco Peña Peña polyclinic in Nuevitas Camagüey.
2- Implement educational intervention and algorithms in relation to basal cell carcinoma.
3. To assess the effectiveness of educational intervention and algorithms in relation to basal cell carcinoma.
The research was carried out using the following methods:

Research methods

A quasi-experimental study was carried out with the population Theoretical level

-Historical-logical, to learn about the evolution and development of scientific knowledge about basal cell carcinoma, as well as the principles that govern its essence.

-Hypothetico-deductive, to construct the hypothesis and infer conclusions.
-Analytical-synthetic, in order to carry out a critical analysis of the documentary sources used, to know the particularities of the object of study and to establish, in a synthetic way, the appropriate interrelation of the elements that make it up.

-Comparative, to establish the analogies and differences of the object of study.

before and after implementing the educational intervention and algorithms.
-Systemic, to consider elements and linkages present in the object of study, in a way that addresses the whole and the parts, with an emphasis on synergies.

From the empirical level:

-Observation, to gather primary information about the patients and the medical care process.
-Measurement, in order to obtain values on the qualities of the object of study, and

process the data obtained through statistical methods.
Quasi-experiment (before-after) without control group, to evaluate the effectiveness

of the educational intervention and the algorithms.

Expected benefits Scientific contribution

• Educational intervention for patients with basal cell carcinoma and the application of the algorithm in patients belonging to the Policlínico Francisco Peña Peña de Nuevitas Camagüey.

An adequate interrelation between the medical actions of the primary and secondary health care levels in tackling the current health problem of basal cell carcinoma.

-Contribution to increasing the knowledge of health care personnel and the general population involved in the medical care of patients in relation to basal cell carcinoma, which will improve their level of professional competence.

-To apply an educational intervention to the study population in relation to basal cell carcinoma, achieving an improvement in their cognitive level.

Social contribution

-Definition of the negative social impact caused by basal cell carcinoma and its complications in the study population.

Enrichment in the application of educational intervention and algorithms in relation to basal cell carcinoma will enable its management and control as well as health education on non-melanocytic skin cancer to patients, families and the general population.

Scientific novelty

The characterisation of patients with basal cell carcinoma was carried out in the critical analysis of the current concepts on the disease that have been referred to in the specialised medical literature, and provides new elements that improve the methods established in Cuba for the treatment, prevention, diagnosis, treatment and follow-up of basal cell carcinoma in this type of cancer and its effects on improving the health of the individual. Educational intervention and the creation of algorithms will enable more comprehensive care for patients who are affected by BCC, which was endorsed, at its core, by a group of expert researchers in the field.

CHAPTER 1

CHARACTERISATION OF BASAL CELL CARCINOMA OR SKIN CANCER IN THE HEALTH AREA

This chapter presents the characterisation of a group of patients with a diagnosis of BCC, belonging to the Francisco Peña Peña polyclinic in Nuevitas, Camagüey, who received medical care.

Objective of the chapter To characterise patients diagnosed with basal cell carcinoma at the Francisco Peña Peña polyclinic in Nuevitas, Camagüey.

Methodological design

A bibliographic review of 59 articles on basal cell carcinoma was carried out for its evaluation and use in the Francisco Peña Peña polyclinic in Nuevitas, Camagüey, during the period from January 2023 to June 2024. The sample consisted of 100 people who met the selection criteria established for the research. Inclusion criteria: Patients with a clinical or histopathological diagnosis of basal cell carcinoma, who belonged, due to their residence, to the areas of the study and exclusion criteria: Patients who could not be interviewed by the author of the research, patients whose clinical history could not be located.

Sample selection criteria

•Inclusion criteria:

Patients with clinical or histopathological diagnosis of basal cell carcinoma, who belonged, due to their residence, to the areas included in the Francisco Peña Peña polyclinic in Nuevitas, Camagüey.

Exclusion criteria:

-Patients who could not be interviewed.

--Patients whose medical records could not be located

-Patients who do not wish to participate

The population participating in the study consisted of 159 patients, 88 female and 71 male, aged between 40 and 80 years, with a high percentage of diabetics, cardiovascular diseases, the most common being high blood pressure, social problems, smoking and coffee,

These patients belong to the municipality of Nuevitas, so it was decided to sample 50 patients with BCC from the main municipality and 50 from the population that wished to participate without suffering from the disease, making the sample significant.

Data collection techniques and procedures In order to identify patients with a diagnosis of basal cell carcinoma, a documentary review was carried out which included: the cancer control register, the register for the histopathological control of malignant neoplasms and the patient care sheets in the different specialities where the different patients are located. These documents, together with the patients' medical records, were used as secondary sources of information. After a critical analysis of the national and international literature specialising in the subject and after consultation with members of the Dermatology Department of the municipality,

CHAPTER 2

BASAL CELL CARCINOMA AS A CURRENT HEALTH PROBLEM

2.1. HISTORY AND CURRENT SITUATION OF BASAL CELL CARCINOMA.

Since ancient times, researchers in world history have referred to non-melanoma skin cancer in dissimilar and controversial ways, and the disease has been conceptualised, described and treated in multiple ways. The earliest reports of BCC date back to studies on ancient Egyptian mummies. During the 14th century it became known as "noli me tangere", meaning "I do not wish you to touch me". (13)

Currently, basal cell carcinoma is defined as a low-grade malignant neoplasm, originating in the cells of the hair follicle and interfollicular areas of the epidermis, invasive and rarely metastatic; however, cases of severe metastasis have been described, resulting in death. Patients with basal cell carcinoma have been found to be more prone to visceral tumours. (14, 15)

Squamous cell carcinoma is conceptualised as an oncoproliferative process of epidermal cells, which retain some characteristics of the normal suprabasal epidermis and has varying degrees of malignancy. Its most important characteristics are anaplasia, rapid growth, local tissue destruction and its ability to metastasise. Numerous factors are involved in the onset of the disease, and its aetiology is therefore diverse. There does not seem to be a single phenomenon responsible, but rather the association of several that over the years lead to the formation of non-melanoma skin cancer. (16)

Ultraviolet radiation is currently known to be the most important cause, mainly in individuals with a genetic predisposition and phenotypic characteristics that make them vulnerable. (17) Ultraviolet A radiation (320-400 nm) is 20 times more abundant than ultraviolet B radiation (290-320 nm) and enhances the deleterious effect of the latter, which has a carcinogenic action 1 600 times greater. Measurements of the ozone layer have shown a decrease in its thickness in the upper strata of the atmosphere, causing ultraviolet radiation reaching the earth's surface to increase considerably in many parts of the planet in recent years. (18)

In the early 20th century, he determined that prolonged exposure to X-rays led to the development of SCC; it was later linked to people who were given Grenz rays as a therapeutic method f o r psoriasis, acne and hirsutism. Squamous cell carcinoma of the lip and mouth is linked to the use of smoked or chewed tobacco, alcohol and betel. HPV infections of serotypes .have been associated with invasive squamous cell carcinoma of the penis, while HPV infection with serotypes 6 and 11 has been documented in verrucous carcinoma. The model par excellence of viral oncogenesis in skin is epidermodysplasia verruciformis, in which HPV serotypes 5 and 8 have been isolated. (14,15,17,19) Actinic keratosis has been identified worldwide as the cutaneous precancerosis with the highest incidence and high tendency to malignant degeneration; it is considered the most frequent and earliest expression of a keratinocyte tumour, although some scientists debate whether it biologically constitutes an intraepithelial carcinoma in situ (a theory promulgated and promoted by Ackerman's group), as some research is inconclusive that all evolve into invasive squamous cell carcinoma. (11,18,21) Bowen's disease is a squamous cell carcinoma located on the skin and mucosa; its aetiology includes significant sun and arsenical exposure, ionising radiation, immunosuppression and HPV infection, especially serotype 16. When it affects the mucosa, mainly that of the penis in uncircumcised males, it is called erythroplasia of Queyrat and exhibits malignant degeneration to invasive squamous cell carcinoma more frequently than Bowen's disease. (22)

Basal cell carcinoma (Annex 5) is subdivided into clinical forms: nodular (most common), ulcerative nodule (ulcus rodens), pigmented, superficial (pagetoid), morpheaform (sclerodermiform or fibrosing) and fibroepithelioma of Pinkus. Associated syndromes such a s nevoid BCC syndrome (Gorlin), unilateral basal cell nevus syndrome and Bazex syndrome have also been described. (23)

Immunosuppression is another factor influencing the occurrence of BCC in anatomical areas unprotected against ultraviolet radiation, e.g. spinocellular carcinoma arising from traumatic scars; some time later, BCC related to burn scars was named "Marjolin's ulcer". In addition, this cutaneous oncoproliferative process has been described in the course of conditions leading to a chronic inflammatory state of the skin such as lichen planus and lichen scleroatrophicus, cutaneous tuberculosis, fungal infections, lupus erythematosus and necrobiosis lipoidica. (20)

Histologically, basal cell carcinomas can be differentiated or undifferentiated, the former differentiating into hairy structures. Hairy structures (keratotic), glands sebaceous glands (sebaceous differentiation) and tubular glands (adenoids), while undifferentiated (solid) ones can be circumscribed or infiltrating; the boundary is not net, because many undifferentiated BCCs have differentiated areas and vice versa. [22,23,24,25] Spinocellular carcinoma has clinical and histopathological features ranging from low malignancy to extremely destructive forms, which is why it has been classified as BCC in situ and invasive or infiltrating BCC (differentiated and undifferentiated); the latter usually develops in 90% of cases from a spinocellular carcinoma in situ located in areas exposed to sunlight. [24,26] With respect to histopathology, squamous cell carcinoma epidermoid is characterised by irregular masses of epidermal cells that proliferate into the dermis and are composed of squamous cells normal yatypical (anaplastic);at the lesions The proportion of atypical cells is higher in poorly differentiated lesions. Differentiation is oriented towards keratinisation which results in the formation of horny pearls. A histological variety with great aggressive and metastasising power has been described, called mucin-producing BCC. [26,27]

Preventive measures to avoid the development of non-melanoma skin cancer are an unrivalled weapon in the fight against the disease. Considering that the marked increase in its incidence is related t o chronic sun exposure, the best preventive measure is to avoid the sun, especially when the intensity of ultraviolet radiation hitting the earth is at its highest (11 - 3 pm). The use of protective clothing such as long-sleeved shirts and trousers, wide-brimmed hats, caps, parasols, dark sunglasses and sunscreens with a sun protection factor of more than 10 % should be insisted upon. Mass screening methods, health promotion and timely treatment of premalignant skin lesions are indispensable measures for prevention. [24, 28,29]

Specific treatment aims primarily at complete removal of the tumour with acceptable cosmetic results; surgical and non-surgical therapeutic modalities are available. Surgical modalities allow histological control of the edges of non-melanoma skin cancer and include excisional methods such as conventional surgery and Mohs micrographic surgery. [25,26,27] Destructive procedures can also be used which, while not allowing histological control of tumour margins, offer the possibility of less invasive and effective treatment of low-risk lesions; these include electrofulguration and curettage, cryosurgery and carbon dioxide laser. [25]

Non-surgical procedures include ionising radiation, which is particularly indicated for patients with tumours located in anatomical areas where surgery is difficult to approach or where surgery inevitably leaves considerable scarring or retraction; photodynamic therapy with aminolevulinic acid, in which the tumour cells to be destroyed are photosensitised by a light source; [26,27,28]

Topical or intralesional 5-fluorouracil chemotherapy; retinoids such as isotretinoin and etretinate;intralesional interferon; and more recently imiquimod, an immunomodulatory drug that possesses antiviral and antitumour activity by inducing the production of cytokines, interleukins, tumour necrosis factor and interferon. [26,29,30, 31,32]The choice of therapeutic procedure will depend on the type of non-melanoma skin cancer, the patient's characteristics and the resources available, while the cosmetic results will depend on the expertise of the treating specialist. The risk of developing another non-melanoma skin cancer within five years of treatment is 35-40%, so it is considered essential that patients once treated are monitored clinically on a regular basis. (33, 34, 35, 36,37)

BCC, also called basal cell epithelioma, is a slow-growing tumour derived from the non-keratinised cells of the epidermal basal layer, and usually develops in photo-exposed areas of individuals with a clear phototype between the third and sixth decade of life. Most are asymptomatic, but there may be invasion into deep layers, recurrences, regional and distant metastases. If left untreated, the tumour progresses to invade subcutaneous tissue, muscle and even bone. It is usually a slow-growing tumour that produces local invasion rather than metastases. [38]

The cause is multifactorial, with intrinsic factors such as age, skin phototype and environmental elements, the best known environmental risk factor being ultraviolet radiation, mainly acute and intermittent exposure.

[39] Several modalities have been described for the treatment of BCC, which broadly fall into two categories: surgical and non-surgical. Radiotherapy, curettage and cryotherapy), thermal destruction (photodynamic therapy), topical (5-fluorouracil), immunomodulatory therapy (topical imiquimod). A selective inhibitor of the Hedgehob signalling pathway (vismodegib) is also indicated. [40] Also in immune modifying therapy are interferons, which have been shown to be effective. None of these treatments is fully effective and all are susceptible to failure in some cases. For these reasons, it is desirable to have an alternative drug treatment that may be more suitable for some patients.

To diagnose skin cancer, the doctor is likely to do the following:

• Examine the skin. The doctor can look at the skin to see if the skin changes are likely to be skin cancer. Further tests may b e needed to confirm the diagnosis.

• Remove a sample of suspicious skin for analysis (skin biopsy). Your doctor may remove suspicious-looking skin for laboratory testing. A biopsy can determine whether you have skin cancer and, if so, what type it is.

Cuba has registered a new drug called "Heberferon" for the treatment of skin cancer, obtained from biotechnological formulations. It is a scientific novelty obtained by the Centre for Genetic Engineering and Biotechnology (CIGB) in Havana after more than 20 years of research and clinical trials.

This injectable medication eliminates or reduces non-melanoma skin tumours and can prevent the after-effects of surgery in areas such as the face where it is difficult to operate, a disease whose main triggering factor is excessive sun exposure, specifically ultraviolet radiation.

The CIGB's production plants have already manufactured more than 10,000 bulbs of the novel drug, which is still under development, in order to evaluate its effectiveness in other types of cancer and the next step is its inclusion in the treatment of other cancers.in the island's basic group of medicines, according to the same source. (40,41) Once diagnosed in its first stage, **HeberFERON®** can be used, which is a pharmaceutical formulation containing a mixture of interferon alpha b2b and interferon in synergistic proportions of anti-tumour activity, it is a safe and effective drug for the treatment of BCC. This treatment is indicated for the treatment of basal cell carcinoma, and as an adjuvant to other treatments, surgical or otherwise, they say they can offer an alternative in those patients who cannot be treated.

Surgical excision is considered the best option for the treatment of BCC, but in patients at high risk or with mutilation criteria, HeberFERON® , a combination containing IFN a2b and IFN and, in synergistic antiproliferative ratios that inhibit tumour cell growth, alone or in combination with other treatments such as radio or chemotherapy, could be considered the best therapeutic option. [42,43]

INFs are a family of polypeptides with pleiotropic functions that are produced by various cells in response to different stimuli, and have potent antiviral properties. INFs have anti-proliferative and anti-cancer activity, directly inhibit tumour cell proliferation and have a more marked inhibitory effect on tumour cells than on normal cells, and are also known to induce apoptosis in some cells, thus not only directly inhibiting tumour cells and destroying them, but also indirectly inhibiting them by stimulating the immune system. (42,43)

At the IGBC where both INFs are produced and with more than a decade of experience in their clinical use and mechanisms of action, Bello,(42) managed to rationally combine both molecules and obtained a more potent anti-tumour effect. These interferons may be the ideal anti-neoplastic treatment, as they exert an apoptotic and anti-proliferative effect, promote anti-angiogenesis and induce immune response.

Thus, in oncology, they are therapeutic options in solid tumours such as melanomas, renal cell carcinoma and AIDS-related Kaposi's sarcoma and have recently been used successfully as first-line or compassionate treatment in osteoblastoma, cervical intraepithelial neoplasia and bladder cancer. (43)

López et al,(44) , in their study, point out that it is important for the patient to have a clinical history, clinical and dermatoscopic examinations of the lesion; It should be explained what the treatment consists of and that a biopsy was necessary to confirm the diagnosis in the event that it was not available, as well as obtaining complementary examinations. It is also clarified that the patient's approval is important and an information sheet should be given to the patient explaining in detail what the treatment consists of.

The authors report that in each session, 3 bulbs (10.5MUI) of HeberFERON® (3.5MUI bulbs) were applied perilesionally and intradermally, 3 times a week for 3 weeks, for a total of 9 doses administered. The patient was followed up every 4 weeks until 16 weeks were completed for the final evaluation, where the size of the lesion, clinical, dermatoscopic and histological changes and adverse events were recorded. To determine the response, the proposed international criteria for the evaluation of response in solid tumours (RECIST) were taken into account, which classifies them as: complete response (CR), When the lesion disappears completely; partial response (PR), if there is a reduction of at least 30 % of the sum of the major diameters; stable disease (SD), when the reduction is not sufficient to classify as partial response; and progressive disease (PD), if there is an increase of at least 20 % in the sum of the major diameters. (44)

The treatment period is variable depending on the treatment scheme chosen. HeberFERON® has its advantages due to its immunomodulatory activity and its potent antiproliferative effect, which is why it has been used safely in Cuba through clinical trials designed by the Centro de Ingeniería Genética y Biotecnología de la Habana (CIGB), in patients with BCC of any size, location and clinical and histological subtype in different hospitals.[13-17] The results of the application of this formulation in the patients in the study were satisfactory. Both reported a minimum of adverse events belonging to the flu-like syndrome such as headache, fever and arthralgia, which disappeared with the application of symptomatic treatment. The tumour was eliminated and good aesthetic and functional results were obtained. [(45)]

If we analyse that there are not only these medicines to treat skin diseases and the importance of their use at international level, other products are developed that can improve the quality of life of these patients, it should be noted that according to the basic pathology of the patients treated with HeberFERON® it was found that 28.57% of the cases studied presented arterial hypertension, followed by those who presented arterial hypertension together with bronchial asthma with 20.4%; which does not coincide with several investigations carried out by different authors.[(46,47)]

Other investigations have shown that the highest percentage of cases also corresponded to this histological subtype of basal cell carcinoma; however, the evolution of each of the BCC subtypes treated with Heberferon should be studied further, as some clinical forms are known to be more aggressive than others, such as basal cell carcinoma with a basosquamous histological subtype. [(48)]

The response to treatment showed that 91.83% of patients treated with HeberFERON® had a complete response to treatment, obtaining a definitive cure in all cases treated. Only 4.08% showed a partial response to treatment, coinciding with multiple studies that have shown a favourable response to treatment with this new drug, a product of Cuban engineering and biotechnology. [(49, 50,51)]

Skin cancer is the most common type of cancer in humans, with basal cell carcinoma being the most common of all skin cancers (80-90%).

%). They rarely metastasise, but can cause significant morbidity and involve younger ages and are successfully treated by surgery, radiotherapy, chemotherapy and cryotherapy, usually at the secondary health care level, however, these treatments are not always possible or desirable. HeberFERON® is a combination of recombinant human alpha and gamma interferons, which has been shown to produce synergistic effects in reducing the proliferation of several cancer cell lines, and has been approved in Cuba for the treatment of basal cell carcinoma. [(43,50)]

The anti-tumour action of interferons (IFNs) is mainly mediated by inhibiting tumour cell growth and inducing tumour cell apoptosis (programmed cell death).

IFNs can arrest tumour growth by differentiation of the tumour cell, they can also act at the cell cycle level where IFN-a targets c-myc, pRB, cyclin D3 and cdc25A genes, controlling apoptosis, IFN-y can exert an antitumour effect, which is dependent on the differentiation state of the cells and the levels of IFN receptors. (50)

HeberFERON® is a synergistic combination of recombinant human alpha 2b and gamma interferons, produced by the Centro de Ingeniería Genética y Biotecnología (CIGB), Havana, Cuba and marketed by Heber Biotec, S.A., the drug is presented in bulbs as a lyophilised powder for injection of 3.5 million international units (MUI), the recommended dose is 10.5 MUI of the powder reconstituted with water for injection, administered 3 times a week for 3 weeks, perilesionally (intradermally) or intralesionally· . (43)

HeberFERON® is a biotechnological product manufactured in Cuba, patented in the Cuban Public Registry of Clinical Trials under code RPCEC00000164.(11) It comes in packs of 10 and 25 2R bulbs with the following composition: recombinant human interferon gamma 0.5 x 106 IU, and recombinant human interferon alpha 2b 3.0 x 106 IU as active ingredients.

Two treatment regimens were used. The first consisted of nine applications of the drug by intradermal and perilesional routes. The injections were administered three times a week, every other day, for three consecutive weeks. The second consisted of 14 intramuscular applications of the preparation, including those patients whose clinical characteristics of the skin and lesions did not allow intradermal and perilesional administration. The doses were injected twice a week for seven weeks.

All patients were evaluated regularly for 16 weeks. At At the end of the follow-up, at week 16, a new dermatoscopic and histopathological study was performed to corroborate the effectiveness of the treatment. (43,50.51) The drug doses were administered after adding one millilitre of water for injection to one bulb of HeberFERON®. In lesions smaller than four centimetres, and in lesions larger than four centimetres, one millilitre of water was added to three bulbs of the biotech product. When the area of the lesion to be treated was larger than four centimetres in diameter, the lesion was imaginatively subdivided into 1.5 cm areas and a dose of one millilitre was administered for each area. If the total dose to be administered was greater than two millilitres, the product was diluted at a ratio of one bulb of drug to 10 ml of water for injection. For lesions smaller than four centimetres, the dose to be administered was administered at equidistant points around the lesion. [43,52,53, 54, 55,56] Drake-Sosa et al.,[57] in 2018 used this treatment, via perilesional infiltration, in patients with basal cell carcinoma; according to their results, the solid and basosquamous subtypes were the most frequent. In the present investigation, solid basal cell carcinomas were most frequently observed.

2.2. FOUNDATIONS FROM THE INTERVENTION EDUCATIONAL INTERVENTION IN RELATION TO BASAL CELL CARCINOMA.

At the present time, we are immersed in a period of reforms in the educational system, linking new technologies and visions of education. In this sense, educational intervention comes to promote events, in order to meet the needs of students.

Educational intervention is understood as a process that encompasses a set of psycho-pedagogical actions, which are designed by experts in the area of intervention, whose objective is to design a programme aimed at solving educational needs. Authors such as Jordán et al. (2011) consider that educational intervention is necessary to promote changes, whether personal, behavioural or knowledge changes, and this is analysed by means of a prior assessment (diagnosis) that provides the basis for the development of an intervention, whose methodology is in line with "change".

It is important to bear in mind that educational intervention goes hand in hand with educational research. In fact, in order to make sense of an intervention, it is necessary to investigate on the basis of previously conducted research, which has studied a series of variables that affect the human being.

In this sense, the main objective of educational intervention is, as the name implies, to intervene in an educational context, in order to support the teaching processes and even the development of the students themselves. Educational interventions aim to influence the academic performance of students.

On the other hand, it is essential to describe that educational intervention is made up of a series of issues, without which it would not be possible to develop a quality intervention. In the following, the aspects that make up an educational intervention are mentioned:

1. Delimitation of the context
2. Needs analysis
3. Justification
4. Objectives
5. Methodology
6. Intervention through sessions
7. Evaluation
8. Conclusions

In this order of ideas, it seems essential to highlight that without the detection of **needs**, it is impossible to develop **educational intervention** projects. In fact, in order to be able to carry out this section, it is essential to carry out a diagnostic process by means of observation itself, specifying the **needs** that must be addressed by means of an **intervention.**

For these reasons, **intervention** becomes essential in education and is positively aligned with the parameters dictated by inclusion. All teachers and schools should promote spaces for **intervention** in the classroom or outside the classroom.

Having said this, it is interesting to note that **educational intervention** in today's society seeks to permeate all new technologies and the tools that derive from them.

However, in order to carry out a quality educational intervention, it is important to bear in mind that it must be the experts who are in charge of carrying out this type of project. The areas of knowledge that deal with these issues are **psycho-pedagogy**, pedagogy and psychology itself. These aspects understand human development in all its dimensions and translate it into the educational sphere, thus promoting quality spaces where intervention is carried out correctly. In this sense, the experts, after delimiting and assessing the needs, concentrate on carrying out a bibliographic research that directs them with key notions related to the perceived needs. Based on this, general and specific objectives are set out, which must be directed to a methodology that helps with the execution of these objectives, by means of activities that are carried out in different sessions and that at the end of them, an overall evaluation of the fulfilment of the objectives is carried out. As a final word, it is important to keep in mind that **educational intervention** is born to support, orient, help and guide people in different environments.It is the intentional action for the realisation and achievement of the integral development of the learner. Educational intervention has a teleological character: there is an agent subject (learner-educator), there is a propositional language (an action is carried out to achieve something), action is taken in order to achieve a future event (the goal) and events are intentionally linked. Educational intervention takes place through processes of self-education and hetero-education, whether formal, non-formal or informal. Educational intervention and pedagogical intervention are not necessarily identified, although in every educational intervention there is a component of pedagogical intervention. This is because no educational action requires a higher level of technical (pedagogical) competence than is necessary to make the goal of the action effective; there are actions that require a low level of technical competence and are effective; there are actions whose level of technical competence has been disseminated and are part of the common heritage of a culture; it is possible to acquire technical competence from one's own practice. The difference between educational intervention and pedagogical intervention is the same as the difference in meaning between the expressions "I know how to do something" and "I know why doing it that way achieves that something and I know what other ways there are to achieve it and I know what needs to be done to redirect the process appropriately". In all these cases there is knowledge of education, but their problem-solving capacity is different. The difference between educational intervention and pedagogical intervention is a conceptual elaboration derived from the advancement of knowledge of education.

For a better development of the research, it was divided into three stages:

1. Diagnostics
2. Intervention.
3. Evaluative.

1. Diagnostic Stage.

Using the Family Clinical Histories, a list was drawn up with names and surnames and addresses of all the families with patients with the disease and possible risks, belonging to the Francisco Peña Peña polyclinic in Nuevitas, Camagüey, who were visited at home where they were asked for informed consent (Appendix 1). They were then given an initial survey (Appendix 2), which was used to collect general data and data related to skin cancer.

2. Intervention stage.

The following characteristics were taken into account in the development of this educational intervention:

Organisational.

The activities were carried out in a room set up for this purpose. Five exchange sessions were designed, with a fortnightly frequency, taking into account that the fifth session was held 3 months after the end of the educational intervention with an approximate duration of 60 minutes; the meeting days were fixed by consensus of the participants.The topics developed in the preparation were related to the felt needs of the participants about the known and unknown aspects of skin cancer, its characteristics, forms of prevention and treatment.At the end of each preparation activity, the participants evaluated themselves through the PNI Technique (Positive, Negative and Interesting Activity), discussing their personal criteria in the Group.

Techniques.

The contents were dealt with in an accessible but still technical language. Terms were defined and exemplification and demonstration were the key actions during the development of each activity. In order to address the participants' lack of knowledge about skin cancer, an intervention with an educational approach was implemented with the following objectives:

- To promote knowledge about skin cancer, as well as the risk factors involved.
- Identify inappropriate behaviours in the population.
- Teach about behaviour and ways to prevent skin cancer, and the short- and long-term consequences of non-compliance.
- To know the myths related to skin cancer.
- Showcase actions dedicated to the prevention of basal cell carcinoma.

• Guidance on the right behaviours to avoid skin cancer and measures to prevent skin cancer from worsening.

2.3. EDUCATIONAL INTERVENTION PROGRAMME. FIRST SESSION.

Theme: Skin cancer. Forms of presentation, symptomatology, causes.

Educational methods.Risk factors.

Objectives:

- To provide information on skin cancer, its fundamental characteristics.
- Reflections on educational methods to prevent skin cancer or the improvement of the disease, its treatment and likelihood of life, knowledge of risk factors.

Organisational Form: Talk - Debate

Time: 60 minutes

Content:

- Concept of skin cancer and classification.
- Different forms of presentation
- Educational methods to be used by families.
- Risk factors in the development of skin cancer
- Alternative treatment and life expectancy.

Aids: Banner, paper, pencil.

Methodology:

Activity 1: Presentation technique. Presentation in pairs.

Activity 2: Brainstorming.

Activity 3: Educational talk on skin cancer, different forms and risk factors.

Activity 4: Group dynamics to discuss educational methods that families can use.

Activity 5: Evaluation and closure activity (PNI).

SECOND SESSION.

Theme: Behaviour of skin cancer patients. Consequences of inappropriate behaviour, in the short and long term.

Objectives:

▶ To teach the fundamental characteristics about the behaviour of patients with skin carcinoma and the psycho-emotional impact on the sufferer.

Organisational Form: Talk - Debate

Time: 50 minutes

Content:

▶ Main behavioural characteristics of patients with skin carcinoma.

▶ Short- and long-term consequences of non-compliance with treatment and preventive measures.

Aids: Banner, paper, pencil.

Methodology:

Activity 1: Summary of the previous session.

Activity 2: Animation technique: Role play.

Activity 3: Educational talk on the characteristics of skin carcinoma and the physical and emotional impact on patients and their families.

Activity 4: Group dynamics to discuss personal experiences.

Activity 5: Evaluation and closure activity (PNI).

THIRD SESSION

Theme: Myths and realities about skin cancer and the implication of not complying with preventive measures or treatment Involvement of society and organisations in society that can help prevent child abuse.

Objectives:

- To reflect on the different myths related to skin cancer.
- To provide knowledge of the different organisations in society that can be involved in skin cancer prevention.

Organisational Form: Talk - Debate

Time: 60 minutes

Content:

- To demonstrate the differences between myths and facts about skin cancer.
- Guiding parental actions to prevent skin cancer.
- Identify the different social sectors that can contribute to the prevention of skin cancer in Cuban society.

Aids: Banner, paper, pencil.

Methodology:

Activity 1: Summary of the previous session.
Activity 3: Participatory technique: Grab your shore.
Activity 4: Evaluation and closing activity (PNI).

FOURTH SESSION

Theme: Preventive measures to avoid non-melanoma skin cancer

Objectives:

- To develop learning skills in the study population.
- Providing knowledge on human protection

Organisational Form: Talk - Debate

Time: 60 minutes

Content:

- Demonstrate the importance of maintaining preventive measures to avoid disease.
- Orient actions aimed at a avoid the suffering fromthe disease.
- Identify the different risk factors.

Aids: Banner, paper, pencil.

Methodology:

Activity 1: Summary of the previous session.
Activity 2: Animation technique: Let's reflect.
Activity 3: Participatory technique: Walk alone and come.
Activity 5: Educational talk on myths related to skin cancer and organisations in society that can be involved in prevention.

FOURTH SESSION

Theme: Characteristics of a patient with skin cancer, its psychological impact and consequences.

Objectives:

- ► To recall the changes that occur in the psychological, social and emotional sphere of a skin cancer patient.
- ► Interpret these changes for the use of this knowledge in everyday life.
- ► Recognise the participation of sectors of society.

Organisational Form: Video - Debate

Time: 60 minutes

Content:

- ► Psychological, emotional and social manifestations in patients with skin cancer.
- ► Linking different sectors in skin cancer prevention.

Aids: TV, video, paper, pencil.

Methodology:

Activity 1: Summary of the previous session.

Activity 2: Presentation of the video related to skin cancer patients .

Activity 3: Group dynamics to discuss the video presented and experiences.

Activity 5: Evaluation and closure technique (PNI).

FIFTH SESSION

Theme: Mass screening methods.

Objectives:

▶ To guide mass screening methods for the diagnosis of non-melanoma skin cancer.

▶ Maintaining health promotion and early treatment of premalignant skin lesions are indispensable measures for prevention.

Organisational Form: Video - Debate

Time: 60 minutes

Content:

▶ Use of protective clothing such as long-sleeved shirts and trousers, wide-brimmed hats, caps, umbrellas, dark sunglasses and sunscreens with sun protection factor.

▶ Mass screening methods, health promotion and early treatment of premalignant skin lesions are indispensable measures for prevention.

Aids: TV, video, paper, pencil.

Methodology:

Activity 1: Summary of the previous session.

Activity 2: Presentation of the video related to the consequences of sun exposure. .

Activity 3: Group dynamics to discuss the video presented and experiences.

Activity 5: Evaluation and closure technique (PNI).

SIXTH SESSION

Topic: Medicinal plants used in the treatment of skin diseases

Objectives:

▶ To guide the practices of biomedicine, self-treatment, and other therapeutic options such as religious therapies and so-called alternatives to traditional treatment.

▶ It guides various traditional medicine practices.

Organisational Form: Video - Debate

Time: 60 minutes

Content:

▶ Medicinal plants have multiple therapeutic applications

▶ The most commonly used plants (Aloe vera, Chamaemelum nobile or Matricaria chamomilla, lemon balm (Melissa offi cinalis L.), theatine (Scoparia dulcis), the stem, leaves and flowers of soursop (Annona muricata), the leaves of the plant called air leaf (Kalanchoe pinnata), the application of ointments from the pulp of avocado (Persea americana), the leaves and flowers of orange (Citrus sinensis L.), bitter tea (Camellia sinensis L.), the rash and skin inflammations are also treated with matico (Buddleja globosa, lam hope).), bitter tea (Camellia sinensis L.), rashes and skin inflammations are also treated with matico (Buddleja globosa, lam hope), Others.

Aids: TV, video, paper, pencil.

Methodology:

Activity 1: Summary of the previous session.

Activity 2: Presentation of the video related to medicinal plants.

Activity 3: Group dynamics to discuss the video presented and experiences.

Activity 5: Evaluation and closure technique (PNI).

3. EVALUATION STAGE.

Three months after the end of the educational intervention, the initial survey was applied to them, in order to check the fixation of the knowledge imparted and their opinion in relation to this educational intervention.

SIXTH SESSION:

Theme: Application of the evaluation survey and participants' opinions of the course.

Objectives:

▶ To assess the knowledge acquired after having received this educational intervention.

▶ Determine the opinion of families regarding the educational intervention.

Methodology:

Activity 1: Application of the evaluation survey.
Activity 2: Participatory technique: The three chairs.
Activity 3: Application of the evaluation technique (PNI).
The following methodological requirements were taken into account for the implementation of both the baseline and endline surveys:

A. The length of the survey was limited to 5 knowledge questions to avoid fatigue.

B. The wording of the introductory material was eloquent and sincere.
C. The questions were designed to be simple, clear, concrete and concise in their formulation.

D. In the choice of words, the vocabulary used and its reference system were taken into account.

E. The questions allowed for only one unambiguous and immediate interpretation.
F. Each question addressed a single idea and dealt with a single topic.
G. Only questions related to the problem in question were asked.
H. Confidential questions were avoided.

A system of theoretical and empirical method, typical of biomedical scientific research, was used, which includes:

Theoretical method: historical-logical method, used as a theoretical foundation on basal cell carcinoma as a background to the research problem.

Documentary analysis method: this was used as a theoretical approach to support the importance of education in this population group, by means of the literature reviewed.

Programme review.

Code of ethics, personal law, legality.

Structural-functional systemic method: based on the variables of knowledge, where different techniques and procedures are put into practice in order to provide care to supposedly healthy people, family and community.

Deduction-induction method: We worked on the basis of the particularities of each person with skin cancer and the others involved, in order to logically identify a reasoning, starting from the particular knowledge to the general and vice versa.

Empirical method: quasi-experimental.

An educational programme was used to identify learning needs based on an initial survey, leading to an evaluative survey, with the aim of assessing the level of knowledge and lifestyle modification and improving the quality of family life.

Techniques used:

1. Remark.
2. Survey.
3. Interview.
4. Test.

Theoretical value: It is given by the theoretical-philosophical and psychological foundation of the education of this group of people, where a planned projection of educational actions was obtained as a result.

CHAPTER 3

ALGORITHMS

The purpose of the algorithms is to make the management of these patients feasible and to achieve quality care, and they will serve as a reference for healthcare institutions.

1.1. ALGORITHM for the implementation of the educational intervention (Annex3)

Objective. To demonstrate the efficacy of an educational intervention for basal cell carcinoma.

The algorithm is developed as an observational framework for educational intervention to the population in relation to basal cell carcinoma, because of the importance of its application will achieve in the study population a level of assimilation of knowledge not only to patients already suffering from the disease but to the population in general, The city of Nuevitas is located north of Camagüey, which is a coastal area and vulnerable to the disease, In recent times the increase of the CBC has taken the interest of the authors to carry out the intervention and that our municipality does not have specialised wards so the patients must travel to the capital city,The algorithm of the educational intervention is a methodological guide for its implementation and desired effect on the cognitive level of the study population. The study was carried out in the Francisco Peña Peña polyclinic in the city of Nuevitas Camagüey, where the problem was identified, with a study population of 100, of whom 59 were diagnosed with BCC and 50 were undiagnosed. An initial survey was carried out to assess the disease, its treatment and level of knowledge.For a better development of the research, it was divided into three stages: Diagnostic, Intervention and Evaluative. For the diagnostic stage, family medical records were used, a list was drawn up with names and surnames and addresses of all the families with patients with the disease and possible risks, belonging to the Francisco Peña Peña polyclinic in Nuevitas, Camagüey, and they were visited at home where they were asked for informed consent. They were then given an initial survey, through which general data and data related to skin cancer were collected.

In the intervention stage, 5 sections were developed with topics related to the CBC of which the topics developed in the preparation were related to the felt needs of the participants, about the known and unknown aspects that they had regarding skin cancer, its characteristics, forms of prevention and treatment. In the evaluation stage at the end of each preparation activity, the participants evaluated themselves through the PNI Technique (Positive, Negative and Interesting of the activity), discussing their personal criteria in the Group.The last section is the closing of the activity which involves various sectors of society and even cultural centres, where various artistic manifestations such as songs, games and paintings will be brought together. In addition, there is coordination with the sales centres of skin products to offer a commercial fair in order to improve the quality of life.

1.2. ALGORITHM FOR THE APPLICATION OF HEBERFERON® FOR THE COMPREHENSIVE CARE OF PATIENTS WITH BASAL CELL CARCINOMA (ANNEX 4).

The application of the Delphi variant of the expert method to establish a consensus on the theoretical and practical basis of the algorithm, despite the fact that our municipality does not carry out the treatment, patients are transferred to specialised centres in Camagüey, an algorithm for the comprehensive care of patients with non-melanoma skin cancer is presented in an argued manner, and the training of the personnel involved in the application of the algorithm is described.

Objectives.

-Establish a consensus on the theoretical and practical basis of the algorithm.

-To specify the guidelines to be followed for the comprehensive care of patients with BCC.

• To increase the level of knowledge about BCC and premalignant skin lesions among health professionals involved in the application of the HeberFERON® algorithm.

Application of the Delphi variant of the expert method General Considerations

In order to establish a consensus on the theoretical and practical foundations of the algorithm, it was decided to consult with experts on elements that were considered essential to the proposal made in this work. These aspects were the following:

-Social need to improve medical care for patients with CBC

- Insufficient dissemination of information about risk factors, aetiology, clinical manifestations and complications of BCC and the application of HeberFERON®.

-The population is poorly informed about risk factors, aetiology and early signs of BCC, and measures are needed to contribute to its prevention and early diagnosis.

-Prioritise screening and treatment of premalignant skin lesions and BCC.

Consider a complete skin examination as essential in the examination of patients with clinical manifestations of BCC, and at-risk individuals and patients should be taught the technique of skin self-examination.

-Early diagnosis of the disease and the use of correct therapeutic methods prevent the development of complications such as: aesthetic and functional disorders, metastasis, perineural infiltration, tumour recurrence and death.

-Determining the level of risk for each tumour (low risk and high risk, complicated or not), according to its clinical and histological characteristics, makes it possible to define the level of medical care where the patient will be treated.

Regular clinical follow-up of patients with BCC after treatment is essential.

-The novelty is centred on the creation of an algorithm for the care of patients with basal cell carcinoma regarding the use of HeberFERON®, based on the deficiencies found in the medical care process for these patients and the current concepts on BCC that have been reflected in the specialised medical literature.

1.3. ALGORITHM FOR THE CARE OF PATIENTS WITH BASAL CELL CARCINOMA.

ALGORITHM CONSTRUCTION

The following definition of algorithm was assumed: an ordered and finite set of operations that allows the solution of a problem to be found. [(58)] To develop the algorithm, a review and analysis of the Guidelines for the diagnosis and treatment of non-melanoma skin cancer was carried out, as well as a review of the national and international medical literature specialising in the subject. As mentioned in the previous section, the theoretical and practical basis of the algorithm was validated by a group of experts in the field.After the algorithm was developed, it was submitted for evaluation to the scientific council of the healthcare institution and the dermatology specialists of the institution. Other specialists were also consulted to validate the research. The suggestions made by the specialists consulted were considered by the authors and the relevant corrections were made; after which, by consensus, the algorithm was approved for use in the research.

FEASIBILITY FOR THE IMPLEMENTATION OF THE ALGORITHMS

With the aim of providing comprehensive care for patients with non-melanoma skin cancer, a series of actions are established for individual, family and community care for patients at the Francisco Peña Peñ4 polyclinic in Nuevitas, Camagüey. These actions are closely interrelated and, for a better understanding, we explain separately the guidelines to be followed in the specialised consultation where patients attend: health promotion, determination of risk groups, dispensation, counselling on lifestyle changes, followed by control or dispensation of cases already diagnosed by means of anamnesis to verify the existence of cutaneous precancerosis and BCC, Patients who come voluntarily to the consultations are referred to the specialist in Dermatology, the specialist carries out a thorough assessment of the skin lesions and provides guidance for complementary examinations, treatment and follow-up in the consultations, or if a non-melanoid carcinoma is reported, a biopsy must be performed and the disease must be reported, When an assessment of the disease is carried out and the specialist determines, according to the specific symptoms, whether it is uncomplicated or complicated, his action is the periodic clinical monitoring of the patients and their referral to other specialised centres for appropriate care and to achieve their recovery or improvement in their general condition through the different specific treatments. Patients diagnosed with a low-risk BCC are given dermatological treatment that includes histopathological studies (conventional surgery or electroconfiguration), follow-up and specialised care. (Annex 5).Efficient health promotion (information, health education and communication) will be carried out by the dermatology specialist or general practitioner, the nursing staff in the health area, and will be aimed at the general population, risk groups, patients and their families. The author considers that informing members of the population about the current health problem of non-melanoma skin cancer and the harm it entails for those affected will help to raise awareness and motivate favourable attitudes.

1.4. ALGORITHM FOR THE TREATMENT OF BASAL CELL CARCINOMA USING HEBERFERON®.

Patients with high and low risk BCC, which are subdivided into primary and recurrent basal cell carcinoma, have a first line conventional treatment which is conventional surgery and micrographic surgery and second line radiotherapy, in patients with BCC it is recommended to follow up to assess recurrence of the treated lesion every four months in the first year, In patients with a history of skin cancer or risk factors for skin cancer, a complete physical examination for the active search of new tumours and recurrence of the treated lesion is recommended every year for life, in primary care services, in patients with a history of skin cancer or risk factors for skin cancer. In patients with a history of skin cancer or risk factors for skin cancer, counselling on the risk of recurrence of the primary lesion and the appearance of new lesions is recommended, as well as education on sun protection measures and skin self-examination, If specific treatments are not used, the characteristics of the cancer are taken into consideration and it is classified to evaluate the possible use of the new product. Once it is diagnosed as a BCC, the specialist will proceed to treat the disease and apply the new HeberFERON® treatment, which is described as follows, it should be noted that this medicine is already used in several countries in the region and even in the USA. (Annex 6)

Form of application:

HeberFERON® is a biotechnological product manufactured in Cuba, patented in the Cuban Public Registry of Clinical Trials with the code RPCEC00000164. It comes in packs of 10 and 25 2R bulbs with the following composition: recombinant human interferon gamma 0.5 x 106 IU, and recombinant human interferon alpha 2b 3.0 x 106 IU as active ingredients. Two treatment regimens were used. The first consisted of nine applications of the drug by intradermal and perilesional routes. The injections were administered three times a week, every other day, for three consecutive weeks. The second consisted of 14 intramuscular applications of the preparation, including those patients whose clinical characteristics of the skin and lesions did not allow intradermal and perilesional administration. Doses were injected twice weekly for seven weeks. All patients were evaluated regularly for 16 weeks. At the end of the follow-up, at week 16, a new dermatoscopic and histopathological study was performed to corroborate the effectiveness of the treatment. The drug doses were administered after adding one millilitre of water for injection to one bulb of HeberFERON®. In lesions smaller than four centimetres, and in lesions larger than four centimetres, one millilitre of water was added to three bulbs of the biotech product. When the area of the lesion to be treated was larger than four centimetres in diameter, the lesion was imaginatively subdivided into 1.5 cm areas and a dose of one millilitre was administered for each area. If the total dose to be administered was greater than two millilitres, the product was diluted at a ratio of one bulb of drug to 10 ml of water for injection. In lesions smaller than four centimetres, the dose to be administered was injected at equidistant points around the lesion. (59) It will be of great interest for dermatology consultations and the application of this novel treatment, which has already been implemented in several countries around the world, with relevant results. In our country it is necessary to train health personnel for the application of the medicine and to achieve its effectiveness. Once the medical treatment has been applied, patients are advised to attend inter-consultation programmes with the specialist.

CONCLUSIONS

The characterisation of patients with basal cell carcinoma assisted in the stage prior to the application of the educational intervention and algorithms revealed insufficient knowledge of these patients and the people involved, including problems with prevention and early diagnosis. An algorithm for the care of patients with basal cell carcinoma was implemented, the theoretical and practical basis of which was validated by the Delphi variant of the expert method. The expected result of the establishment of the algorithm demonstrated its effectiveness in improving the process of medical care for patients with basal cell carcinoma, as comprehensive care for these patients was guaranteed, with the occurrence of few complications.

BIBLIOGRAPHICAL REFERENCES

1. Choi Y, Byun J, Choi J, Jung J. Identification of predictive variables for the recurrence of oral mucocele. Med Oral Patol Oral and Oral Cir 2019; 24:0-0.

2. Lee YJ, Kwon JG, Han HH. Surgical deroofing in the treatment of patients with atrial pseudocyst. Auris Nasus Larynx 2018.doi:10.1016/j.anl.2018.10.017.

3. Braun RP, Ludwig S, Marghoob AA. Differential Diagnosis of Seborrheic Keratosis: Clinical and Dermoscopic Features. J Drugs Dermatol 2017; 16:835-42.

4. Morse DC, Tschen JA, Silapunt S. Atrophic dermatofibroma in an elderly male - a rarely described variant of a common lesion. Dermatol Online J 2018; 24.URL http://www.ncbi.nlm.nih.gov/pubmed/30142716

5. Koh U, Janda M, Aitken JF, et al. 'Mind your Moles' study: protocol of a prospective cohort study of melanocytic naevi. BMJ Open 2018; 8:e025857.

6. Dominguez-Cruz J, Ruiz-Villaverde R. The '5R + R' Rule: A simple and comprehensive method for diagnosis of actinic keratosis. Sultan Qaboos Univ Med J 2019; 19:e81-2.

7. Ministry of Public Health (CUB). Independent Cancer Control Section. Prevention, diagnosis and treatment of skin cancer [Internet]. La Havana: Editorial Ciencias Médicas,2023. Available at: http:/ / w w w . bvscuba.sld.cu/libro/prevencion-diagnostico-y-tratamiento-del- skin-cancer/

8. Martínez-Guerra EC, Sánchez-Uriarte ME, Medina-Bojórquez A, Torres S, Alcalá-Pérez D. Skin cancer in patients younger than 40 years. Dermatol Rev Mex [internet]. Jan. 2017 [cited 28 Jun. 20];61(1):[approx. 7 p.]. Available at: http://www.medigraphic.com/pdfs/derrevmex/rmd- 2017/rmd171b.pdf.

9. Roque Pérez L, Alfonso Alfonso Y. About the article: Educational intervention aimed at sun protection in children. Rev 16 April [internet]. 2018 [cited 6 Jun. 2024];57(268):[approx. 3 p.]. Available from: http://www.rev16deabril.sld.cu/index.php/16_04 /article/view/661/pdf_170

10. Ministry of Public Health. Anuario Estadístico de Salud 2017. Havana: National Directorate of Medical Records and Health Statistics; 2018.

11. González R. R. Cáncer de piel, asunto a seguir [internet]. Vanguardia. 3 Feb. 2018; Sect. Villa Clara [cited 17 Dec. 2024]. Available from:

http://www.vanguardia.cu/villa-clara/10745 -cancer-of-skin-issue-to-follow.
12. Requena C, Alsina M, Morgado-Carrasco D, et al. Kaposi's sarcoma and cutaneous angiosarcoma: guidelines for diagnosis and treatment. Actas Dermosifiliogr 2018; 109:878-87.
13. Lebbe C, Garbe C, Stratigos AJ, et al. Diagnosis and treatment of Kaposi's sarcoma: European consensus-based interdisciplinary guideline (EDF/EADO/EORTC). Eur J Cancer 2019; 114:117-27.
14. Dañino-García M, Domínguez-Cruz JJ, Pérez-Ruiz C, et al. Clinical-epidemiological characteristics of Merkel cell carcinoma in a series of 38 patients. Actas Dermosifiliogr 2019; 110:360-5.
15. Llombart B, Kindem S, Chust M. Update on Merkel cell carcinoma: key imaging techniques, prognostic factors, treatment and follow-up. Actas Dermosifiliogr 2017; 108:98-107.
16. Soleymani T, Aasi SZ, Novoa R, Hollmig ST. Atypical Fibroxanthoma and Pleomorphic Dermal Sarcoma: Updates on Classification and Management. Dermatol Clin 2019; 37:253-9.
17. Chapman LW, Yu SS, Arron ST. Atypical Fibroxanthoma. Semin Cutan Med Surg 2019; 38:E65-6.
18. Sarac E, Yuksel M, Turkmen IC, Ozdemir M. Case for diagnosis. Atypical fibroxanthoma. An Bras Dermatol 2019; 94:239-41.
19. Merritt BG, Degesys CA, Brodland DG. Extramammary Paget disease. Dermatol Clin 2019; 37:261-7.
20. Falto-Aizpurua L, Seyfer S, Krishnan B, Orengo I. Cutaneous metastasis of a pulmonary carcinoid tumour. Cutis 2017; 99:E13-5.
21. Watts CG, Cust AE, Menzies SW, Mann GJ, Morton RL. Cost- Effectivenessof Skin Surveillance Through a Specialized Clinic for Patients at High Riskof Melanoma. J Clin Oncol. 2017 Jan;35(1):63-71.
22. Moscarella E, Tion I, Zalaudek I, Lallas A, Kyrgidis A, Longo C, et al. Bothshort-term and long-term dermoscopy monitoring is useful in detectingmelanoma in patients with multiple atypical nevi. J Eur Acad DermatolVenereol. 2017 Feb;31(2):247-51.
23. Smedinga H, Verkouteren JAC, Steyerberg EW et al. Occurrence of metachronous basal cell carcinomas: a prognostic model. Br J Dermatol. 2017 Oct; 177(4):1113-1121.

24. Tejera-Vaquerizo A, Descalzo-Gallego M, Otero-Rivas M, Posada-García C, Rodríguez-Pazos L, Pastushenko I et al. Incidence and mortality of skin cancer in Spain: systematic review and meta-analysis. 2017.
25. Paucar K. Six cases of skin cancer detected in EsSalud campaign [Internet]. Página3. 2017 [Cited 13 Nov. 2022]. Available from: http:// pagina3.pe/detectan-seis-casos-de-cancer-de-piel-en-campana-de- essalud.
26. T. J. Brinker et al., 'Deep learning outperformed 136 of 157 dermatologists in a head-to-head dermoscopic melanoma image classification task', Eur. J. Cancer, vol. 113, pp. 47-54, May 2019, doi: 10.1016/j.ejca.2019.04.001.
27. M. A. Marchetti et al., 'Results of the 2016 International Skin Imaging Collaboration International Symposium on Biomedical Imaging challenge: Comparison of the accuracy of computer algorithms to dermatologists for the diagnosis of melanoma from dermoscopic images', J. Am. Acad. Dermatol. vol. 78, no. 2. Feb. 2018, doi: 10.1016/j.jaad.2017.08.016.1016/j.ejca.2019.05.023.
28. H. A. Haenssle et al., 'Man against machine: diagnostic performance of a deep learning convolutional neural network for dermoscopic melanoma recognition in comparison to 58 dermatologists', Ann. Oncol. vol. 29, no. 8, Aug. 2018, doi: 10.1093/annonc/mdy166.
29. Department of Dermatology, The Warren Alpert Medical School, Brown University, Providence, RI, USA et al., 'Epidemiology of Melanoma', in Cutaneous Melanoma: Etiologyand Therapy, Department of Surgical Oncology, Fox Chase Cancer Center, Philadelphia,PA, USA, W. H. Ward, J. M. Farma, and Department of Surgical Oncology, Fox Chase Cancer Center, Philadelphia,PA, USA, Eds. Codon Publications, 2017. doi: 10.15586/codon.cutaneousmelanoma.2017.ch1.
30. C. Garbe et al., 'Time trends in incidence and mortality of cutaneous melanoma in Germany', J. Eur. Acad. Dermatol. Venereol., vol. 33, no. 7. Jul. 2019, doi: 10.1111/jdv.15322.
31. Martínez-Guerra EC, Sánchez-Uriarte ME, Medina-Bojórquez A, Torres S, Alcalá-Pérez D. Skin cancer in patients younger than 40 years. Dermatol Rev Mex [internet]. Jan. 2017 [cited 28 Dec. 2022];61(1):[approx.7p.]. Available at: http://www.medigraphic.com/pdfs/derrevmex/rmd- 2017/rmd171b.pdf.
32. González RR. Skin cancer, an issue to follow [Internet]. Vanguardia. 3 Feb. 2018; Sect. Villa Clara [Cited 17 Dec. 2022]. Available at: http://www.vanguardia.cu/villa-

clara/10745-cancer-de-piel-asunto-a-seguir
33. Dias da Silva R, Inácio Dias MA. Incidence of basal cell and squamous cell carcinoma in patients treated in a cancer hospital. REFACS. 2017; 5(2):228-34.
34. Iribarren BO, Ramírez SM, Madariaga GJA, Riveros FO, Valdés VC, Toledo SJ. Basal and squamous cell carcinoma of the skin. Case series. Rev Chil Cir [Internet]. 2018 [Cited 2 Dec. 2022]; 70(4): [approx. 6 p]. Available at: https://scielo.conicyt.cl/scielo.php?script=sci_arttext&pid=S0718-40262018000400315&lng=es
35. NIH National Cancer Institute. Skin Cancer Treatment (PDQ®) - Patient Version. [Internet]. [Cited 2 Dec. 2022] **Available from** https://www.cancer.gov/espanol/tipos/piel/paciente/tratamiento-piel-pdq.

36. Clínic Barcelona. Treatment of skin cancer [Internet]. 2018.[cited 16 Jan 2023]. Available at .https://www.clinicbarcelona.org/asistencia/enfermedades/cancer-de-skin/treatment

37. May Click. Skin cancer. [Internet]. 2018 [cited 16 Jan 2023 Available at https://www.mayoclinic.org/es-es/diseases-conditions/skin- cancer/diagnosis-treatment/drc-20377608.
38. Alcalá Pérez D, Carmona Contreras FP, González Gutiérrez JF. Aggressive basal cell carcinoma. Dermatology CMQ. [Internet]. 2018[Cited 14 Dec. 2022]; 16(2):134-137.
39. Bernia E, Llombart B, Serra-Guillén B, Bancalari E, Nagore E, Requena C, et al. Experience with vismodegib in advanced basal cell carcinoma in a cancer centre. Actas dermosifiliogr. [Internet].2018 [Cited 14 Dec. 2022]; 109(9):813-820.
40. Adachi K, Yoshida Y, Noma H, Goto H, Yamamoto O. Characteristics of multiple basal cell carcinomas: The first study on Japanese patients. J Dermatol. [Internet].2018 [Cited 14 Dec. 2022]; 45(10):1187-1190.
41. Castellano Maturell G, Nápoles Pastoriza DD, Niebla Chávez R, Berenguer Gouarnaluses M, Sánchez Álvarez JE. HeberFERON(R) in the treatment of basal cell carcinoma. Case report. Rev April 16 [Internet]. 2019 [Cited 14 Dec. 2022]; 58(271): [approx. 3p]. Available from: https://www.rev16deabril.sld.cu/index.php/16_04/article/view/776

42. Bello Rivero I. A Synergistic immunotherapy for skin cancer. Health and Medicine 2017 [accessed:14/05/2019].Available at: http://www.scientia.global/professor-iraldo-

bello-rivero-synergistic- immunotherapy-skin-cancer/
43. Bello I, García Y, Duncan Y, Vázquez D, Santana H, Besada V, et al. HeberFERON, a new formulation of IFNs with improved pharmacodynamics: Perspective for cancer treatment. Seminars in Oncology. 2018;45:27-33. DOI: https://doi.org/10.1053/j.seminoncol.2018.04.007

44. López-Pupo N, Manganelly-Fonseca Y, Tablada-Robinet M, Jacas-Portuondo A, Girón-Maturell Y. Usefulness of HeberFERON® in patients with basal cell carcinoma. **MEDISAN** [Internet]. 2021 [cited 24 Jan 2023]; 25(6):[approx.11p.].Available at: https://medisan.sld.cu/index.php/san/article/view/3867

45. Rojas Rondón I, Duncan Roberts Y, Gómez Cabrera C G, Ramírez García L K, Vigoa Aranguren L, Hernández Rodríguez R, Tuero Iglesias A, Bello Rivero I. Heberferon administration in palpebral basal cell carcinoma in 2 cases. Available from: http://dx.doi.org/10.21931/RB/2016.01.02.6

46. Fuentes Mederos L, Mayo Abad O, Hidalgo Guerrero IL, Paz Pérez Z, Márquez Bravo D. Introduction and consistency of Heberferon production at the Parenteral Products Plant 3. RTQ [Internet]. 2018 [Cited 12 Dec. 2022]; 38(3):[approx. 13 p].Available from: http://scielo.sld.cu/pdf/rtq/v38n3/rtq12318.pdf

47. Piña Rodríguez Y, Piña Russinyol JJ, Piña Rodríguez JJ, Castro Morillo AM, Darias Domínguez C. Dermatoscopy to establish minimal surgical margins in the resection of basal cell carcinomas. Rev Med Electron [online]. 2018 [Cited 2 Dec, 2022]; 40(1):[approx. 9 p]. Available from: http://scielo.sld.cu/scielo.php?script=sci_arttext&pid=S1684-18242018000100012&lng=en.

48. Darias Domínguez C, Garrido Celis J. Basal cell carcinoma. A current challenge for the dermatologist. Rev Med Electron [online]. 2018 [Cited 21 Dec. 2022]; 40(1):[Approx.10p].Available at: http:/ / www.revmedicaelectronica.sld.cu/index.php/rme/article/view/2498/370 7

49. Rodríguez-Fonseca R, de-la-Rosa-Santana J, López-Wilson A, Santiesteban-Puerta S, Cabrera-Pérez C. Treatment with Heberferon in patients with basal cell carcinoma at the Hospital Docente Clínico Quirúrgico "Dr. Miguel Enríquez", Havana. Gaceta Médica Estudiantil [Internet]. 2020 [cited 17 Jan 2023]; 1 (2):[approx. 10 p.]. Available from: https://revgacetaestudiantil.sld.cu/index.php/gme/article/view/30

50. López Pupo Natacha, Manganelly Fonseca Yarien, Tablada Robinet María Elena,

Jacas Portuondo Ana Lucía, Girón Maturell Yaimaris. Utility of Heberferon® in patients with basal cell carcinoma. MEDISAN [Internet].2021Dec [cited2023Jan 17];25(6): 1297-1308. Available from: http://scielo.sld.cu/scielo.php?script=sci_arttext&pid=S1029-30192021000601297&lng=en. Epub 03-Nov-2021.
51. Fahradyan A, Howell A, Wolfswinkel E, Tsuha M, Sheth P, Wong A. Updates on the management of non-melanoma skin cancer (NMSC). Healthcare. 2017[Cited 7 Dec. 2022]; 5(82):1-24. Available from: https://doi:10.3390/healthcare5040082
52. Bordelois-Abdo JA, López-Mateus M, Fernández-Ramírez I, Lagos-Ordóñez KJ. Characterisation of the older adult patient with a probable diagnosis of skin cancer. Rev. inf. sci. [Internet]. Feb 2019 [cited 3 Nov. 2023]; 97(4):7-16. Available from: http://scielo.sld.cu/pdf/ric/v98n1/1028-9933-ric- 98-01-7.pdf.
53. Sánchez-Linares V, Rodríguez-Montagne D, Cifuentes-Suárez JP, Román-Simón M, Pérez-García C, Bello-Rivero I. Gorlin-Goltz syndrome. A case report. Gac Méd Espirit [Internet]. Dec 2018 [cited 8 Nov. 2022]; 20(3):136-45. Available from: http://scielo.sld.cu/pdf/gme/v20n3/1608- 8921-gme-20-03-136.pdf.
54. Anasagasti-Angulo L, García-Vega Y, Collazo S, Jiménez-Barbán Y, Tijerino-Arrieta E, Ballester-Caballero Y, et al. HeberFERON, formulation based on IFNs alpha2b and gamma for the treatment of non-melanoma skin cancer. AMJ [Internet]. 2017 [Cited 1 Nov. 2022]; 10(6):509-15. Available from: https://www.researchgate.net/profile/Yanelda_Garcia/publication/318191920 HeberFERON_formulation_based_on_IFNs_alpha2b_and_gamma_for_the_treatment _of_non- melanoma_skin_cancer/links/5a58ca64aca2727d60814ca3/HeberFERON-formulation-based-on-IFNs-alpha2b-and-gamma-for-the-treatment-of-non- melanoma-skin-cancer.pdf
55. Fernández-Martori M, Bello-Rivero I, Duncan-Roberts Y. Treatment of basal cell carcinoma with interferons alpha-2b and gamma in primary care. MEDICC Rev [Internet]. 2018 [Cited 6 Dec.2022];20(1):11-17. Available from: https://www.scielosp.org/pdf/medicc/2018.v20n1/11-17/en
56. Roque-Pérez L, González-Escudero M. HeberFERON: an effective solution for basal cell carcinoma. Rev. Electron. Zoilo [Internet]. 2019 [cited 2 Dec. 2022]; 44(3):[approx. 11 p.]. Available from: http://revzoilomarinello.sld.cu/index.php/zmv/article/download/1713/pdf_589
57. Drake-Sosa DV, Rojas-Barlys L. HeberFERON in patients with basal cell

carcinoma treated in the municipality of Puerto Padre, Las Tunas. Rev. Electron. Zoilo [Internet]. 2018 [Cited 7 Dec. 2022]; 43(6):[approx. 5 p.].Available in: http://www.revzoilomarinello.sld.cu/index.php/zmv/article/download/1573/pdf _531

58. Dictionary of the Spanish language. 21st ed. Madrid: Espasa Calpe; 1994. Algoritmo; p.99.

59. CECMED. Summary rom of the characteristicsof the product. HeberFERON®. Available at: https:/ / www.cecmed.cu/sites/default/files/adjuntos/rcp/biologicos/rcp_heberf eron

ANNEXES

Annex 1

INFORMED CONSENT

I, give my approval to participate in the research that will be carried out to characterize a group of patients with non-melanoma skin cancer and those who wish to participate in order to achieve a knowledge of the population about it, in the Francisco Peña Peña polyclinic in Nuevitas. It has been explained to me that my participation is voluntary and if I do not accept or if I withdraw from the study when I consider it appropriate, my name will not be divulged. This research is only carried out for research purposes. For the record and of my own free will, I sign this informed consent together with the doctor who gave me the explanations, on this day of the month of the year

Signature of doctor

Signature of patient

Annex 2

Survey.

Good afternoon

Today we are going to conduct an anonymous survey to test your knowledge about skin cancer, this research is voluntary for those who wish to participate and to reach the conclusion to apply an educational intervention and algorithms to increase the knowledge about skin cancer4 and its treatment.

Eda Sex

1. What do you understand by skin cancer?
2. What risk factors are you aware of that cause skin cancer?
3. What protective measures are you aware of?
4. How would you implement any protection?
5. If you suffer from the disease, you are aware of the medical treatment. If NO Which ones?
6. You receive information about the disease from the health centres.Yes No

Annex 3

Algorithm for applying educational intervention to the population in relation to basal cell carcinoma.

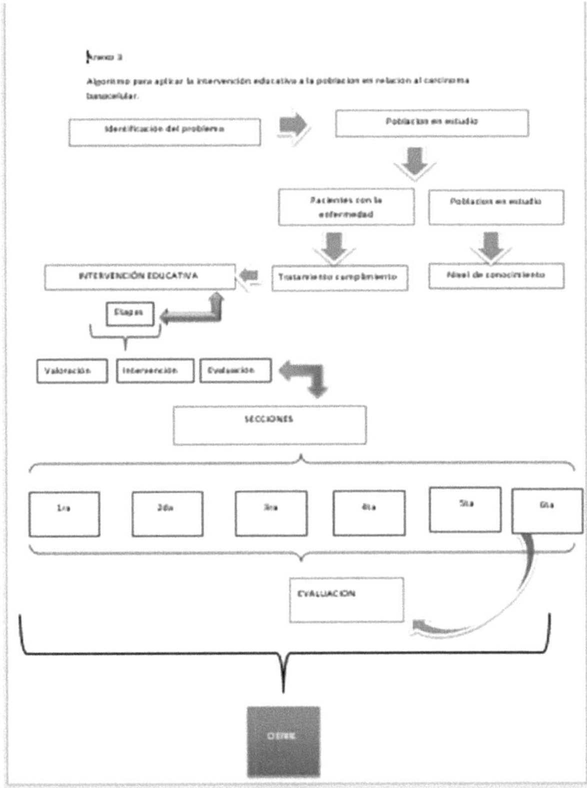

Annex 4

Expert consultation questionnaire

All the consultations that follow refer to studies to improve the process of medical care for patients with basal cell carcinoma, characterising these patients who belong to the study areas determined that there are difficulties not only in the management, control and treatment but also in the study population of the disease. Please express your opinion on the following, marking with an X what you select for your opinion.

1-There is a social need to improve medical care for patients with basal cell carcinoma due to the notable increase in the number of people who arrive at the clinic in an advanced stage of the disease, with significant functional and aesthetic alterations, leading to varying degrees of disability and in some cases death.

Adequate Inadequate

2. The level of dissemination of information on risk factors, aetiology, clinical manifestations and complications of skin cancer or basal cell carcinoma in the mass media, hospital billboards, polyclinics and family doctor's offices is insufficient and needs to be increased.

Adequate Inadequate

3- If the population is aware of the risk factors, aetiological factors and incipient signs of basal cell carcinoma or skin cancer, it will be able to adopt measures that contribute to its prevention and early diagnosis.

Adequate Inadequate

4-In persons at risk, early detection and treatment of lesions with HeberFERON is essential.

Adequate Inadequate

5-The examination of the patient should include a complete skin examination and skin self-examination should be taught.

Adequate Inadequate

6. Do you believe that early diagnosis of the disease prevents complications in these patients?

Adequate Inadequate

7. The determination of the level of tumour risk (low risk and high risk, complicated or not) makes it possible to decide on the level of medical care where patients will be treated with HeberFERON.

Adequate Inadequate

8. Regular clinical follow-up of patients after treatment is essential.

Adequate Inadequate

9. The novelty is centred on the creation of an algorithm for the comprehensive care of patients with basal cell carcinoma through the application of HeberFERON and its effectiveness in treatment, based on the inadequacies found in medical care and the different definitions of it.

Adequate Inadequate

Annex 5

Algorithm for the comprehensive care of patients with basal cell carcinoma.

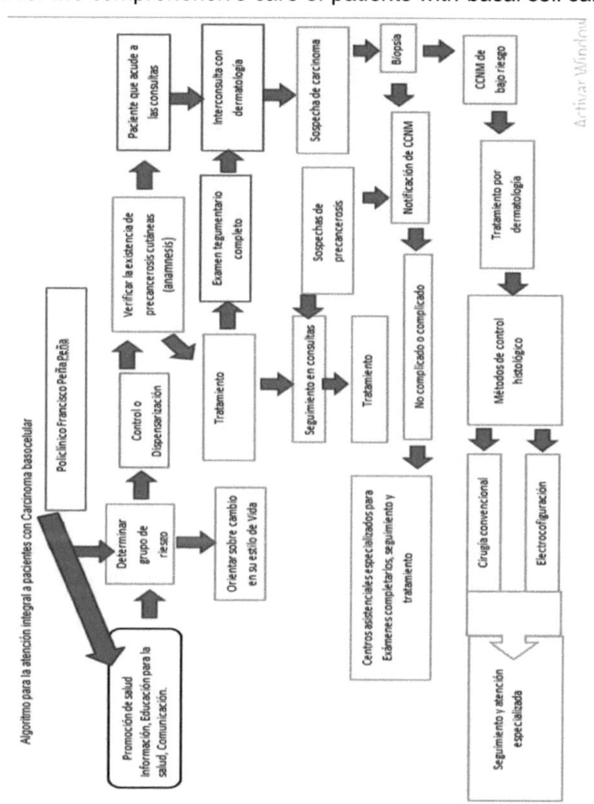

Annex 6

Algorithm for the treatment of basal cell carcinoma using HeberFERON®.

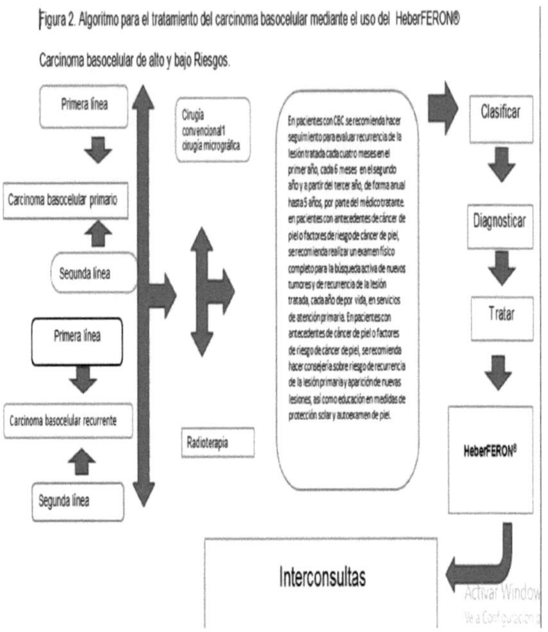

AUTHORS

Roger Rios Escobar Leydis Suárez Ramos Milaris Cabreja Heredia

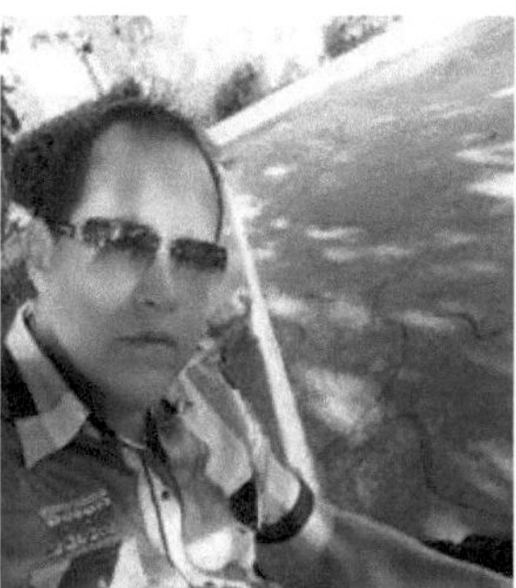

Roger Rios Escobar, specialised in paediatric intensive care, assistant professor, researcher with experience in teaching and research. He has published in international journals and has participated in health events and is currently collaborating with the prestigious Spanish academic publishing house.

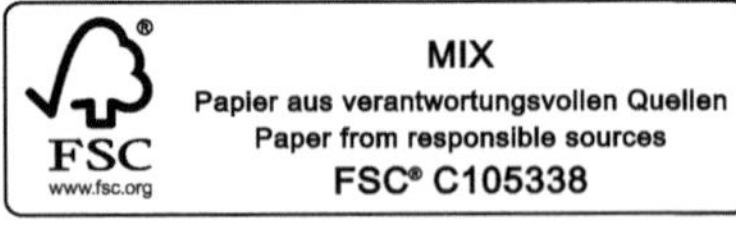

Printed by Books on Demand GmbH, Norderstedt / Germany